Fertility & Conception JOURNAL

THIS BOOK BELONGS TO:

_____

How to Use

Whether you have been trying for a while, or you are now taking a new step, this book is designed to help give you a complete picture of your cycle while tracking symptoms of ovulation, helping you to time sex with your partner perfectly and get pregnant quicker. If you are concerned that you may not be ovulating, or are having trouble conceiving, this record may provide valuable insight and give you information to take when you visit the doctor.

Fertility Window

Sperm live around five days when in the right kind of cervical mucus in a woman's body. Eggs can only be fertilized for about 24 hours after being released from your ovary. Therefore, your "fertile window" is typically considered the day of ovulation and the five days prior. However, your chance of getting pregnant goes up significantly if you have sex the day or 2 prior to ovulation and on ovulation day. While the "average" day of ovulation is on cycle day 14, this varies greatly among women. It is important to be familiar with your own symptoms of ovulation in order to increase the liklihood that you will time intercourse so that egg and sperm can meet.

Cycle Tracking

Begin by tracking your cycle on the logbook pages. The day you begin bleeding is cycle day 1. Once you have tracked a full cycle and estimated your ovulation date, you will be able to count how many days after ovulation it was until you started your next period. This is usually around 12-14 days and is called your luteal phase. If you are having trouble figuring out when you ovulated, counting back 12-14 days from when you began your period is a good way to get a starting point of estimation. If your cycles are irregular or very long, it is even more important to track symptoms of ovulation to maximize your chances of pregnancy each cycle. If you have doctor appointments or need to take notes, makes lists, or journal, there are beautiful pages for that in the back of this book.

Terms + Definitions

CD = Cycle Day : The day you begin your period is CD 1. The average cycle length is 28 days, but cycles consistently ranging from 21 to 40 days can be considered normal.

DPO = Days Past Ovulation : Knowing how many DPO you are will help determine when you are able to take a pregnancy test to see if you are pregnant this cycle.

CM = Cervical Mucus : Understanding the types of cervical mucus can help you to predict where you are in your cycle and how close ovulation is. This is an important part of identifying when you are fertile. You can check the consistency of what comes off on the toilet paper when you wipe, or you may have to use clean hands to reach up to your cervix for a sample. Use your fingers to feel and determine the consistency.

> **Dry**: No secretions, not fertile

> **Sticky**: Thick, pasty, crumbly or gummy secretions; low fertility

> **Creamy**: Like a lotion; you are *nearing or in your fertility window*

> **Wet**: Transparent, thin secretions; you are *nearing or in your fertility window*

> **Egg White**: The consistency of egg whites and sometimes can be stretched far between fingers; *this is your most fertile time*

IC = Intercourse : IC is the abbreviation used when charting to indicate sex when trying to conceive.

LH = Luteinizing Hormone : A rise in this hormone signals release of the egg. At home ovulation tests measure LH.

Ovulation Test : A positive ovulation test typically means that you should ovulate within the next 24 to 36 hours. Your best chance to conceive is in the first 2-3 days following a positive test. While these tests can be costly, you don't have to test every day. If you choose to use these tests, you will typically begin testing a few days before you typically ovulate. Always read the information that comes with your particular test and follow it for best results.

Follicular Phase : The time between the first day of your period and ovulation. Estrogen rises and the egg is being prepared for release.

Luteal Phase : The time between ovulation and when your period begins. The lining of your uterus gets thicker preparing for a possible pregnancy. If there is no pregnancy, it will shed after the luteal phase, beginning a new cycle.

BBT = Basal Body Temperature : Your waking temperature. This has been used for generations to monitor fertility. However, tracking BBT requires a commitment and does nothing to help predict ovulation. A rise in BBT indicates and confirms that you did ovulate. By the time this is indicated, it is too late to conceive. Therefore, there is not a place to chart BBT in this journal, but if you are unsure if you are ovulating, there is space under notes to chart this daily if needed.

YOU'LL NEVER BE "READY" *start anyway*

Example

*actual log has room for cycles up to 40 days

CD	DATE	CM / FLOW	LH	OV	IC	DPO	NOTES
1	8/27	heavy					
2	8/28	heavy					
3	8/29	medium					meds
4	8/30	medium					
5	8/31	medium					
6	9/1	light					
7	9/2	light					
8	9/3	sticky	−				
9	9/4	creamy	−				
10	9/5	creamy	+		✓		
11	9/6	wet					
12	9/7	egg white		✓	✓	0	ovulation pain
13	9/8	sticky				1	
14	9/9					2	
15						3	
16						4	
17						5	
18						6	
19						7	
20						8	
21						9	
22						10	
23						11	breast tenderness & bloating
24						12	– PMS or pregnancy?
25		spotting				13	pregnancy test negative
26	9/21	heavy				14	cd 1
27							

Pick up med refill Monday morning!

♥ CYCLE LENGTH _25 days_

♥ OVULATION ON CD _12_

♥ FOLLICULAR PHASE LENGTH _11_

♥ LUTEAL PHASE LENGTH _13_

Cycle Log 🖤

CD	DATE	CM / FLOW	LH	OV	IC	DPO	NOTES
1							
2							
3							
4							
5							
6							
7							
8							
9							
10							
11							
12							
13							
14							
15							
16							
17							
18							
19							
20							
21							
22							
23							
24							
25							
26							
27							
28							
29							
30							

CM = dry, sticky, creamy, wet, egg white   FLOW = heavy, medium, light, spotting

CD	DATE	CM / FLOW	LH	OV	IC	DPO	NOTES
31							
32							
33							
34							
35							
36							
37							
38							
39							
40							

♥ CYCLE LENGTH _____

♥ OVULATION ON CD _____

♥ FOLLICULAR PHASE LENGTH _____

♥ LUTEAL PHASE LENGTH _____

Cycle Log

CD	DATE	CM / FLOW	LH	OV	IC	DPO	NOTES
1							
2							
3							
4							
5							
6							
7							
8							
9							
10							
11							
12							
13							
14							
15							
16							
17							
18							
19							
20							
21							
22							
23							
24							
25							
26							
27							
28							
29							
30							

CM = dry, sticky, creamy, wet, egg white   FLOW = heavy, medium, light, spotting

CD	DATE	CM / FLOW	LH	OV	IC	DPO	NOTES
31							
32							
33							
34							
35							
36							
37							
38							
39							
40							

❤ CYCLE LENGTH _____

❤ OVULATION ON CD _____

❤ FOLLICULAR PHASE LENGTH _____

❤ LUTEAL PHASE LENGTH _____

Cycle Log ♥

CD	DATE	CM / FLOW	LH	OV	IC	DPO	NOTES
1							
2							
3							
4							
5							
6							
7							
8							
9							
10							
11							
12							
13							
14							
15							
16							
17							
18							
19							
20							
21							
22							
23							
24							
25							
26							
27							
28							
29							
30							

CM = dry, sticky, creamy, wet, egg white   FLOW = heavy, medium, light, spotting

CD	DATE	CM / FLOW	LH	OV	IC	DPO	NOTES
31							
32							
33							
34							
35							
36							
37							
38							
39							
40							

❤ CYCLE LENGTH_____

❤ OVULATION ON CD _____

❤ FOLLICULAR PHASE LENGTH _____

❤ LUTEAL PHASE LENGTH _____

Cycle Log

CD	DATE	CM / FLOW	LH	OV	IC	DPO	NOTES
1							
2							
3							
4							
5							
6							
7							
8							
9							
10							
11							
12							
13							
14							
15							
16							
17							
18							
19							
20							
21							
22							
23							
24							
25							
26							
27							
28							
29							
30							

CM = dry, sticky, creamy, wet, egg white   FLOW = heavy, medium, light, spotting

CD	DATE	CM / FLOW	LH	OV	IC	DPO	NOTES
31							
32							
33							
34							
35							
36							
37							
38							
39							
40							

❤ CYCLE LENGTH _____

❤ OVULATION ON CD _____

❤ FOLLICULAR PHASE LENGTH _____

❤ LUTEAL PHASE LENGTH _____

Cycle Log

CD	DATE	CM / FLOW	LH	OV	IC	DPO	NOTES
1							
2							
3							
4							
5							
6							
7							
8							
9							
10							
11							
12							
13							
14							
15							
16							
17							
18							
19							
20							
21							
22							
23							
24							
25							
26							
27							
28							
29							
30							

CM = dry, sticky, creamy, wet, egg white   FLOW = heavy, medium, light, spotting

CD	DATE	CM / FLOW	LH	OV	IC	DPO	NOTES
31							
32							
33							
34							
35							
36							
37							
38							
39							
40							

❤ CYCLE LENGTH _____

❤ OVULATION ON CD _____

❤ FOLLICULAR PHASE LENGTH _____

❤ LUTEAL PHASE LENGTH _____

Cycle Log ♥

CD	DATE	CM / FLOW	LH	OV	IC	DPO	NOTES
1							
2							
3							
4							
5							
6							
7							
8							
9							
10							
11							
12							
13							
14							
15							
16							
17							
18							
19							
20							
21							
22							
23							
24							
25							
26							
27							
28							
29							
30							

CM = dry, sticky, creamy, wet, egg white   FLOW = heavy, medium, light, spotting

CD	DATE	CM / FLOW	LH	OV	IC	DPO	N O T E S
31							
32							
33							
34							
35							
36							
37							
38							
39							
40							

❤ CYCLE LENGTH_____

❤ OVULATION ON CD _____

❤ FOLLICULAR PHASE LENGTH _____

❤ LUTEAL PHASE LENGTH _____

Cycle Log ♥

CD	DATE	CM / FLOW	LH	OV	IC	DPO	NOTES
1							
2							
3							
4							
5							
6							
7							
8							
9							
10							
11							
12							
13							
14							
15							
16							
17							
18							
19							
20							
21							
22							
23							
24							
25							
26							
27							
28							
29							
30							

CM = dry, sticky, creamy, wet, egg white   FLOW = heavy, medium, light, spotting

CD	DATE	CM / FLOW	LH	OV	IC	DPO	NOTES
31							
32							
33							
34							
35							
36							
37							
38							
39							
40							

❤ CYCLE LENGTH _____

❤ OVULATION ON CD _____

❤ FOLLICULAR PHASE LENGTH _____

❤ LUTEAL PHASE LENGTH _____

Cycle Log ♥

CD	DATE	CM / FLOW	LH	OV	IC	DPO	NOTES
1							
2							
3							
4							
5							
6							
7							
8							
9							
10							
11							
12							
13							
14							
15							
16							
17							
18							
19							
20							
21							
22							
23							
24							
25							
26							
27							
28							
29							
30							

CM = dry, sticky, creamy, wet, egg white   FLOW = heavy, medium, light, spotting

CD	DATE	CM / FLOW	LH	OV	IC	DPO	NOTES
31							
32							
33							
34							
35							
36							
37							
38							
39							
40							

❤ CYCLE LENGTH _____

❤ OVULATION ON CD _____

❤ FOLLICULAR PHASE LENGTH _____

❤ LUTEAL PHASE LENGTH _____

Cycle Log

CD	DATE	CM / FLOW	LH	OV	IC	DPO	NOTES
1							
2							
3							
4							
5							
6							
7							
8							
9							
10							
11							
12							
13							
14							
15							
16							
17							
18							
19							
20							
21							
22							
23							
24							
25							
26							
27							
28							
29							
30							

CM = dry, sticky, creamy, wet, egg white   FLOW = heavy, medium, light, spotting

CD	DATE	CM / FLOW	LH	OV	IC	DPO	N O T E S
31							
32							
33							
34							
35							
36							
37							
38							
39							
40							

❤ CYCLE LENGTH _____

❤ OVULATION ON CD _____

❤ FOLLICULAR PHASE LENGTH _____

❤ LUTEAL PHASE LENGTH _____

Cycle Log

CD	DATE	CM / FLOW	LH	OV	IC	DPO	NOTES
1							
2							
3							
4							
5							
6							
7							
8							
9							
10							
11							
12							
13							
14							
15							
16							
17							
18							
19							
20							
21							
22							
23							
24							
25							
26							
27							
28							
29							
30							

CM = dry, sticky, creamy, wet, egg white   FLOW = heavy, medium, light, spotting

CD	DATE	CM / FLOW	LH	OV	IC	DPO	NOTES
31							
32							
33							
34							
35							
36							
37							
38							
39							
40							

❤ CYCLE LENGTH _____

❤ OVULATION ON CD _____

❤ FOLLICULAR PHASE LENGTH _____

❤ LUTEAL PHASE LENGTH _____

Cycle Log

CD	DATE	CM / FLOW	LH	OV	IC	DPO
1						
2						
3						
4						
5						
6						
7						
8						
9						
10						
11						
12						
13						
14						
15						
16						
17						
18						
19						
20						
21						
22						
23						
24						
25						
26						
27						
28						
29						
30						

NOTES

CM = dry, sticky, creamy, wet, egg white   FLOW = heavy, medium, light, spotting

CD	DATE	CM / FLOW	LH	OV	IC	DPO	NOTES
31							
32							
33							
34							
35							
36							
37							
38							
39							
40							

❤ CYCLE LENGTH _____

❤ OVULATION ON CD _____

❤ FOLLICULAR PHASE LENGTH _____

❤ LUTEAL PHASE LENGTH _____

Cycle Log ♥

CD	DATE	CM / FLOW	LH	OV	IC	DPO	NOTES
1							
2							
3							
4							
5							
6							
7							
8							
9							
10							
11							
12							
13							
14							
15							
16							
17							
18							
19							
20							
21							
22							
23							
24							
25							
26							
27							
28							
29							
30							

CM = dry, sticky, creamy, wet, egg white   FLOW = heavy, medium, light, spotting

CD	DATE	CM / FLOW	LH	OV	IC	DPO	NOTES
31							
32							
33							
34							
35							
36							
37							
38							
39							
40							

❤ CYCLE LENGTH _____

❤ OVULATION ON CD _____

❤ FOLLICULAR PHASE LENGTH _____

❤ LUTEAL PHASE LENGTH _____

Cycle Log

CD	DATE	CM / FLOW	LH	OV	IC	DPO	NOTES
1							
2							
3							
4							
5							
6							
7							
8							
9							
10							
11							
12							
13							
14							
15							
16							
17							
18							
19							
20							
21							
22							
23							
24							
25							
26							
27							
28							
29							
30							

CM = dry, sticky, creamy, wet, egg white   FLOW = heavy, medium, light, spotting

CD	DATE	CM / FLOW	LH	OV	IC	DPO	NOTES
31							
32							
33							
34							
35							
36							
37							
38							
39							
40							

♥ CYCLE LENGTH _____

♥ OVULATION ON CD _____

♥ FOLLICULAR PHASE LENGTH _____

♥ LUTEAL PHASE LENGTH _____

Cycle Log

CD	DATE	CM / FLOW	LH	OV	IC	DPO	NOTES
1							
2							
3							
4							
5							
6							
7							
8							
9							
10							
11							
12							
13							
14							
15							
16							
17							
18							
19							
20							
21							
22							
23							
24							
25							
26							
27							
28							
29							
30							

CM = dry, sticky, creamy, wet, egg white   FLOW = heavy, medium, light, spotting

CD	DATE	CM / FLOW	LH	OV	IC	DPO	NOTES
31							
32							
33							
34							
35							
36							
37							
38							
39							
40							

❤ CYCLE LENGTH _____

❤ OVULATION ON CD _____

❤ FOLLICULAR PHASE LENGTH _____

❤ LUTEAL PHASE LENGTH _____

Cycle Log

CD	DATE	CM / FLOW	LH	OV	IC	DPO	NOTES
1							
2							
3							
4							
5							
6							
7							
8							
9							
10							
11							
12							
13							
14							
15							
16							
17							
18							
19							
20							
21							
22							
23							
24							
25							
26							
27							
28							
29							
30							

CM = dry, sticky, creamy, wet, egg white   FLOW = heavy, medium, light, spotting

CD	DATE	CM / FLOW	LH	OV	IC	DPO	N O T E S
31							
32							
33							
34							
35							
36							
37							
38							
39							
40							

❤ CYCLE LENGTH _____

❤ OVULATION ON CD _____

❤ FOLLICULAR PHASE LENGTH _____

❤ LUTEAL PHASE LENGTH _____

Cycle Log

CD	DATE	CM / FLOW	LH	OV	IC	DPO	NOTES
1							
2							
3							
4							
5							
6							
7							
8							
9							
10							
11							
12							
13							
14							
15							
16							
17							
18							
19							
20							
21							
22							
23							
24							
25							
26							
27							
28							
29							
30							

CM = dry, sticky, creamy, wet, egg white   FLOW = heavy, medium, light, spotting

CD	DATE	CM / FLOW	LH	OV	IC	DPO	N O T E S
31							
32							
33							
34							
35							
36							
37							
38							
39							
40							

♥ CYCLE LENGTH _____

♥ OVULATION ON CD _____

♥ FOLLICULAR PHASE LENGTH _____

♥ LUTEAL PHASE LENGTH _____

Cycle Log

CD	DATE	CM / FLOW	LH	OV	IC	DPO	NOTES
1							
2							
3							
4							
5							
6							
7							
8							
9							
10							
11							
12							
13							
14							
15							
16							
17							
18							
19							
20							
21							
22							
23							
24							
25							
26							
27							
28							
29							
30							

CM = dry, sticky, creamy, wet, egg white   FLOW = heavy, medium, light, spotting

CD	DATE	CM / FLOW	LH	OV	IC	DPO	NOTES
31							
32							
33							
34							
35							
36							
37							
38							
39							
40							

❤ CYCLE LENGTH_____

❤ OVULATION ON CD _____

❤ FOLLICULAR PHASE LENGTH _____

❤ LUTEAL PHASE LENGTH _____

Cycle Log ♥

CD	DATE	CM / FLOW	LH	OV	IC	DPO	NOTES
1							
2							
3							
4							
5							
6							
7							
8							
9							
10							
11							
12							
13							
14							
15							
16							
17							
18							
19							
20							
21							
22							
23							
24							
25							
26							
27							
28							
29							
30							

CM = dry, sticky, creamy, wet, egg white   FLOW = heavy, medium, light, spotting

CD	DATE	CM / FLOW	LH	OV	IC	DPO	NOTES
31							
32							
33							
34							
35							
36							
37							
38							
39							
40							

❤ CYCLE LENGTH _____

❤ OVULATION ON CD _____

❤ FOLLICULAR PHASE LENGTH _____

❤ LUTEAL PHASE LENGTH _____

Cycle Log

CD	DATE	CM / FLOW	LH	OV	IC	DPO	NOTES
1							
2							
3							
4							
5							
6							
7							
8							
9							
10							
11							
12							
13							
14							
15							
16							
17							
18							
19							
20							
21							
22							
23							
24							
25							
26							
27							
28							
29							
30							

CM = dry, sticky, creamy, wet, egg white   FLOW = heavy, medium, light, spotting

CD	DATE	CM / FLOW	LH	OV	IC	DPO	NOTES
31							
32							
33							
34							
35							
36							
37							
38							
39							
40							

💜 CYCLE LENGTH _____

💜 OVULATION ON CD _____

💜 FOLLICULAR PHASE LENGTH _____

💜 LUTEAL PHASE LENGTH _____

Cycle Log

CD	DATE	CM / FLOW	LH	OV	IC	DPO	NOTES
1							
2							
3							
4							
5							
6							
7							
8							
9							
10							
11							
12							
13							
14							
15							
16							
17							
18							
19							
20							
21							
22							
23							
24							
25							
26							
27							
28							
29							
30							

CM = dry, sticky, creamy, wet, egg white   FLOW = heavy, medium, light, spotting

CD	DATE	CM / FLOW	LH	OV	IC	DPO	NOTES
31							
32							
33							
34							
35							
36							
37							
38							
39							
40							

❤ CYCLE LENGTH _____

❤ OVULATION ON CD _____

❤ FOLLICULAR PHASE LENGTH _____

❤ LUTEAL PHASE LENGTH _____

Cycle Log

CD	DATE	CM / FLOW	LH	OV	IC	DPO	NOTES
1							
2							
3							
4							
5							
6							
7							
8							
9							
10							
11							
12							
13							
14							
15							
16							
17							
18							
19							
20							
21							
22							
23							
24							
25							
26							
27							
28							
29							
30							

CM = dry, sticky, creamy, wet, egg white   FLOW = heavy, medium, light, spotting

CD	DATE	CM / FLOW	LH	OV	IC	DPO	N O T E S
31							
32							
33							
34							
35							
36							
37							
38							
39							
40							

♥ CYCLE LENGTH _____

♥ OVULATION ON CD _____

♥ FOLLICULAR PHASE LENGTH _____

♥ LUTEAL PHASE LENGTH _____

Cycle Log ♥

CD	DATE	CM / FLOW	LH	OV	IC	DPO	NOTES
1							
2							
3							
4							
5							
6							
7							
8							
9							
10							
11							
12							
13							
14							
15							
16							
17							
18							
19							
20							
21							
22							
23							
24							
25							
26							
27							
28							
29							
30							

CM = dry, sticky, creamy, wet, egg white   FLOW = heavy, medium, light, spotting

CD	DATE	CM / FLOW	LH	OV	IC	DPO	N O T E S
31							
32							
33							
34							
35							
36							
37							
38							
39							
40							

♥ CYCLE LENGTH _____

♥ OVULATION ON CD _____

♥ FOLLICULAR PHASE LENGTH _____

♥ LUTEAL PHASE LENGTH _____

Cycle Log ♥

CD	DATE	CM / FLOW	LH	OV	IC	DPO	NOTES
1							
2							
3							
4							
5							
6							
7							
8							
9							
10							
11							
12							
13							
14							
15							
16							
17							
18							
19							
20							
21							
22							
23							
24							
25							
26							
27							
28							
29							
30							

CM = dry, sticky, creamy, wet, egg white   FLOW = heavy, medium, light, spotting

CD	DATE	CM / FLOW	LH	OV	IC	DPO	NOTES
31							
32							
33							
34							
35							
36							
37							
38							
39							
40							

♥ CYCLE LENGTH _____

♥ OVULATION ON CD _____

♥ FOLLICULAR PHASE LENGTH _____

♥ LUTEAL PHASE LENGTH _____

Cycle Log

CD	DATE	CM / FLOW	LH	OV	IC	DPO	NOTES
1							
2							
3							
4							
5							
6							
7							
8							
9							
10							
11							
12							
13							
14							
15							
16							
17							
18							
19							
20							
21							
22							
23							
24							
25							
26							
27							
28							
29							
30							

CM = dry, sticky, creamy, wet, egg white   FLOW = heavy, medium, light, spotting

CD	DATE	CM / FLOW	LH	OV	IC	DPO	NOTES
31							
32							
33							
34							
35							
36							
37							
38							
39							
40							

❤ CYCLE LENGTH _____

❤ OVULATION ON CD _____

❤ FOLLICULAR PHASE LENGTH _____

❤ LUTEAL PHASE LENGTH _____

Cycle Log

CD	DATE	CM / FLOW	LH	OV	IC	DPO	NOTES
1							
2							
3							
4							
5							
6							
7							
8							
9							
10							
11							
12							
13							
14							
15							
16							
17							
18							
19							
20							
21							
22							
23							
24							
25							
26							
27							
28							
29							
30							

CM = dry, sticky, creamy, wet, egg white   FLOW = heavy, medium, light, spotting

CD	DATE	CM / FLOW	LH	OV	IC	DPO	NOTES
31							
32							
33							
34							
35							
36							
37							
38							
39							
40							

♥ CYCLE LENGTH_____

♥ OVULATION ON CD _____

♥ FOLLICULAR PHASE LENGTH _____

♥ LUTEAL PHASE LENGTH _____

Cycle Log

CD	DATE	CM / FLOW	LH	OV	IC	DPO	NOTES
1							
2							
3							
4							
5							
6							
7							
8							
9							
10							
11							
12							
13							
14							
15							
16							
17							
18							
19							
20							
21							
22							
23							
24							
25							
26							
27							
28							
29							
30							

CM = dry, sticky, creamy, wet, egg white   FLOW = heavy, medium, light, spotting

CD	DATE	CM / FLOW	LH	OV	IC	DPO	NOTES
31							
32							
33							
34							
35							
36							
37							
38							
39							
40							

❤ CYCLE LENGTH _____

❤ OVULATION ON CD _____

❤ FOLLICULAR PHASE LENGTH _____

❤ LUTEAL PHASE LENGTH _____

Cycle Log

CD	DATE	CM / FLOW	LH	OV	IC	DPO	NOTES
1							
2							
3							
4							
5							
6							
7							
8							
9							
10							
11							
12							
13							
14							
15							
16							
17							
18							
19							
20							
21							
22							
23							
24							
25							
26							
27							
28							
29							
30							

CM = dry, sticky, creamy, wet, egg white   FLOW = heavy, medium, light, spotting

CD	DATE	CM / FLOW	LH	OV	IC	DPO	NOTES
31							
32							
33							
34							
35							
36							
37							
38							
39							
40							

❤ CYCLE LENGTH _____

❤ OVULATION ON CD _____

❤ FOLLICULAR PHASE LENGTH _____

❤ LUTEAL PHASE LENGTH _____

Cycle Log ♥

CD	DATE	CM / FLOW	LH	OV	IC	DPO	NOTES
1							
2							
3							
4							
5							
6							
7							
8							
9							
10							
11							
12							
13							
14							
15							
16							
17							
18							
19							
20							
21							
22							
23							
24							
25							
26							
27							
28							
29							
30							

CM = dry, sticky, creamy, wet, egg white   FLOW = heavy, medium, light, spotting

CD	DATE	CM / FLOW	LH	OV	IC	DPO	NOTES
31							
32							
33							
34							
35							
36							
37							
38							
39							
40							

♥ CYCLE LENGTH _____

♥ OVULATION ON CD _____

♥ FOLLICULAR PHASE LENGTH _____

♥ LUTEAL PHASE LENGTH _____

Cycle Log

CD	DATE	CM / FLOW	LH	OV	IC	DPO	NOTES
1							
2							
3							
4							
5							
6							
7							
8							
9							
10							
11							
12							
13							
14							
15							
16							
17							
18							
19							
20							
21							
22							
23							
24							
25							
26							
27							
28							
29							
30							

CM = dry, sticky, creamy, wet, egg white   FLOW = heavy, medium, light, spotting

CD	DATE	CM / FLOW	LH	OV	IC	DPO	NOTES
31							
32							
33							
34							
35							
36							
37							
38							
39							
40							

❤ CYCLE LENGTH _____

❤ OVULATION ON CD _____

❤ FOLLICULAR PHASE LENGTH _____

❤ LUTEAL PHASE LENGTH _____

Cycle Log

CD	DATE	CM / FLOW	LH	OV	IC	DPO	NOTES
1							
2							
3							
4							
5							
6							
7							
8							
9							
10							
11							
12							
13							
14							
15							
16							
17							
18							
19							
20							
21							
22							
23							
24							
25							
26							
27							
28							
29							
30							

CM = dry, sticky, creamy, wet, egg white   FLOW = heavy, medium, light, spotting

CD	DATE	CM / FLOW	LH	OV	IC	DPO	N O T E S
31							
32							
33							
34							
35							
36							
37							
38							
39							
40							

❤ CYCLE LENGTH _____

❤ OVULATION ON CD _____

❤ FOLLICULAR PHASE LENGTH _____

❤ LUTEAL PHASE LENGTH _____

Cycle Log

CD	DATE	CM / FLOW	LH	OV	IC	DPO	NOTES
1							
2							
3							
4							
5							
6							
7							
8							
9							
10							
11							
12							
13							
14							
15							
16							
17							
18							
19							
20							
21							
22							
23							
24							
25							
26							
27							
28							
29							
30							

CM = dry, sticky, creamy, wet, egg white   FLOW = heavy, medium, light, spotting

CD	DATE	CM / FLOW	LH	OV	IC	DPO	NOTES
31							
32							
33							
34							
35							
36							
37							
38							
39							
40							

❤ CYCLE LENGTH _____

❤ OVULATION ON CD _____

❤ FOLLICULAR PHASE LENGTH _____

❤ LUTEAL PHASE LENGTH _____

Cycle Log

CD	DATE	CM / FLOW	LH	OV	IC	DPO	NOTES
1							
2							
3							
4							
5							
6							
7							
8							
9							
10							
11							
12							
13							
14							
15							
16							
17							
18							
19							
20							
21							
22							
23							
24							
25							
26							
27							
28							
29							
30							

CM = dry, sticky, creamy, wet, egg white   FLOW = heavy, medium, light, spotting

CD	DATE	CM / FLOW	LH	OV	IC	DPO	N O T E S
31							
32							
33							
34							
35							
36							
37							
38							
39							
40							

❤ CYCLE LENGTH _____

❤ OVULATION ON CD _____

❤ FOLLICULAR PHASE LENGTH _____

❤ LUTEAL PHASE LENGTH _____

Notes + Journaling

....
....
....
....
....
....
....
....
....
....
....
....
....
....
....
....
....
....
....
....
....
....
....
....
....

Notes + Journaling

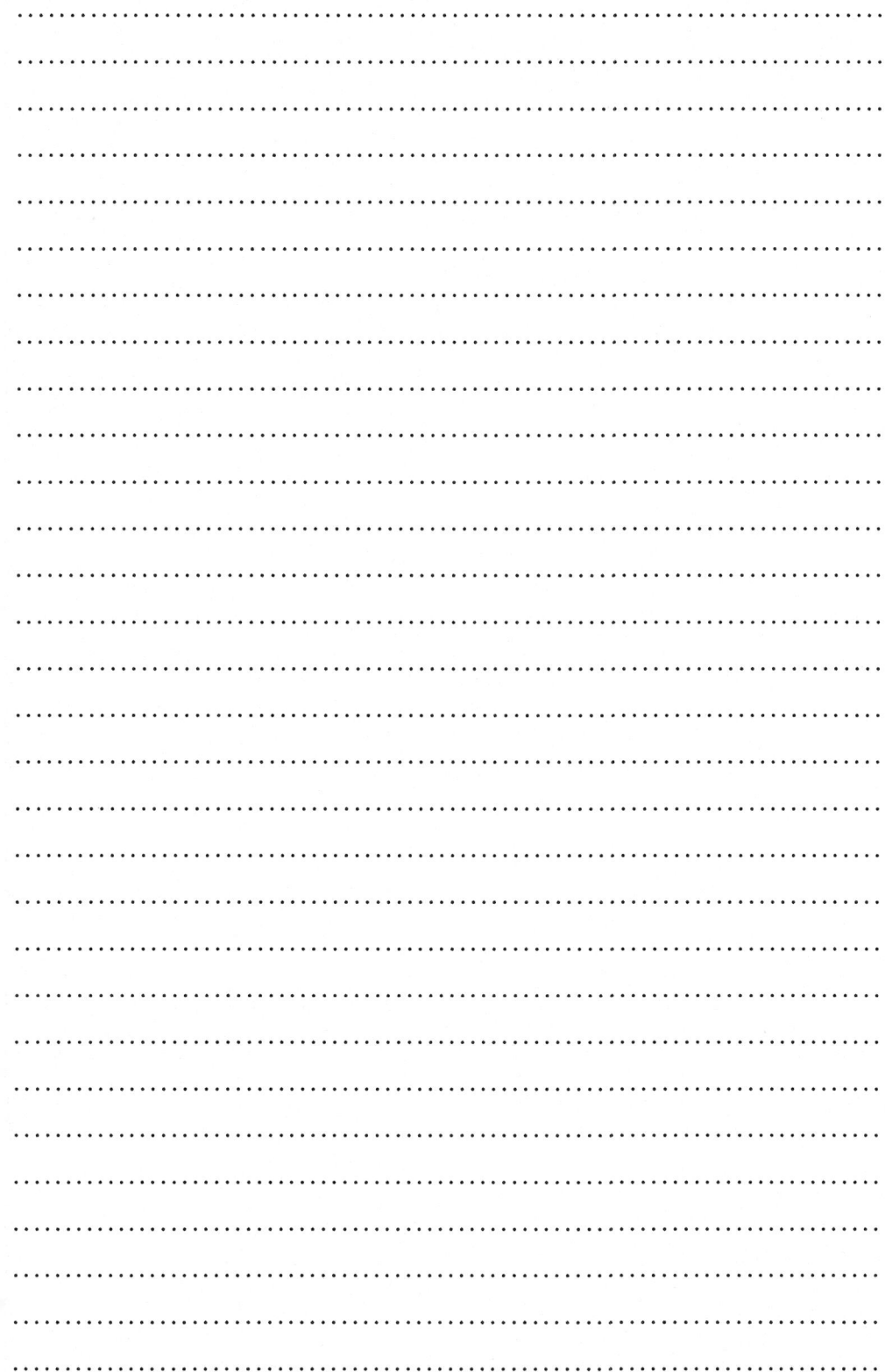

Notes + Journaling

....

....

....

....

....

....

....

....

....

....

....

....

....

....

....

....

....

....

....

....

....

....

....

....

....

Notes + Journaling

Notes + Journaling

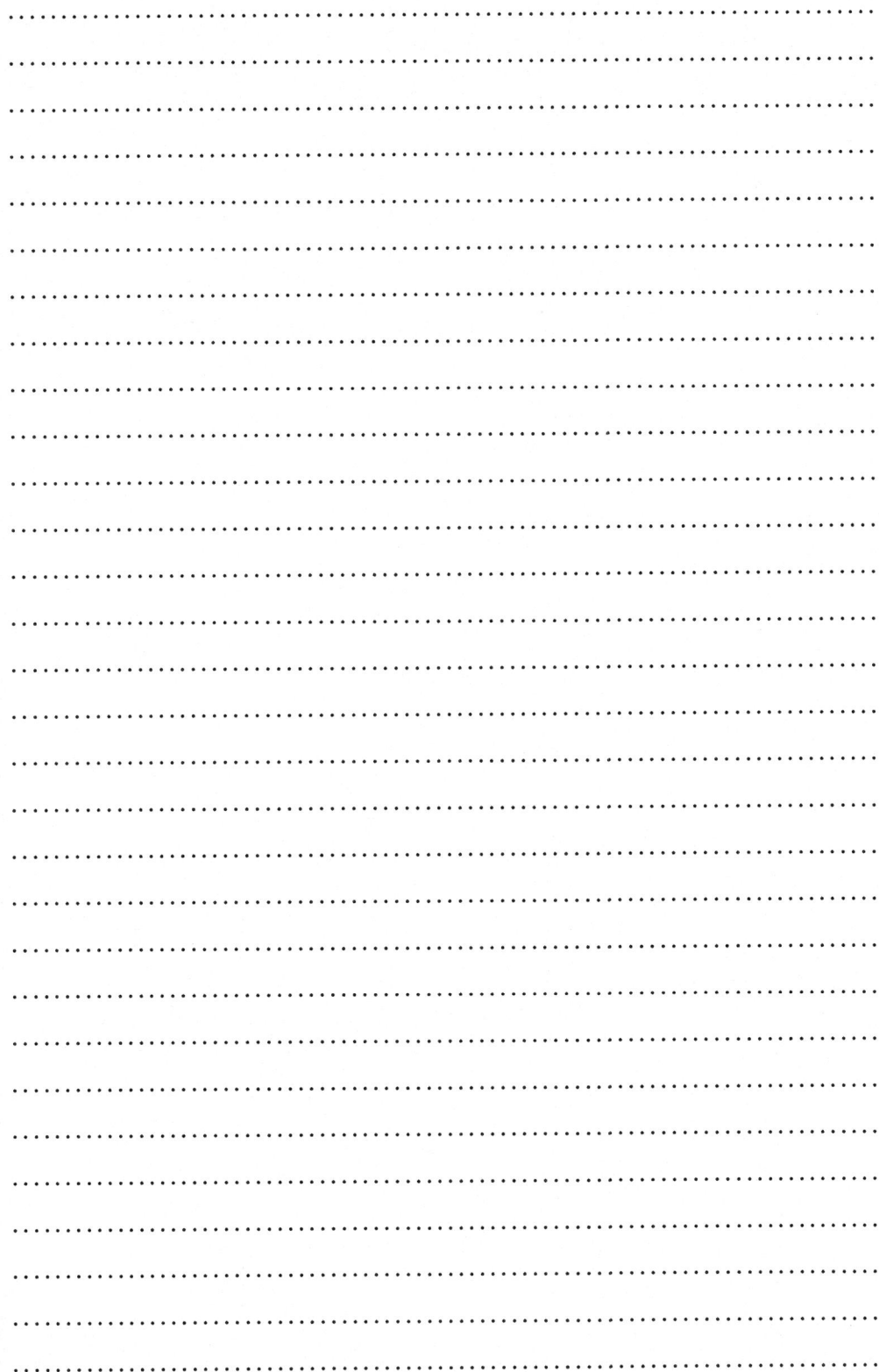

Notes + Journaling

....

....

....

....

....

....

....

....

....

....

....

....

....

....

....

....

....

....

....

....

....

....

....

....

....

....

Notes + Journaling

Notes + Journaling

Notes + Journaling

Notes + Journaling

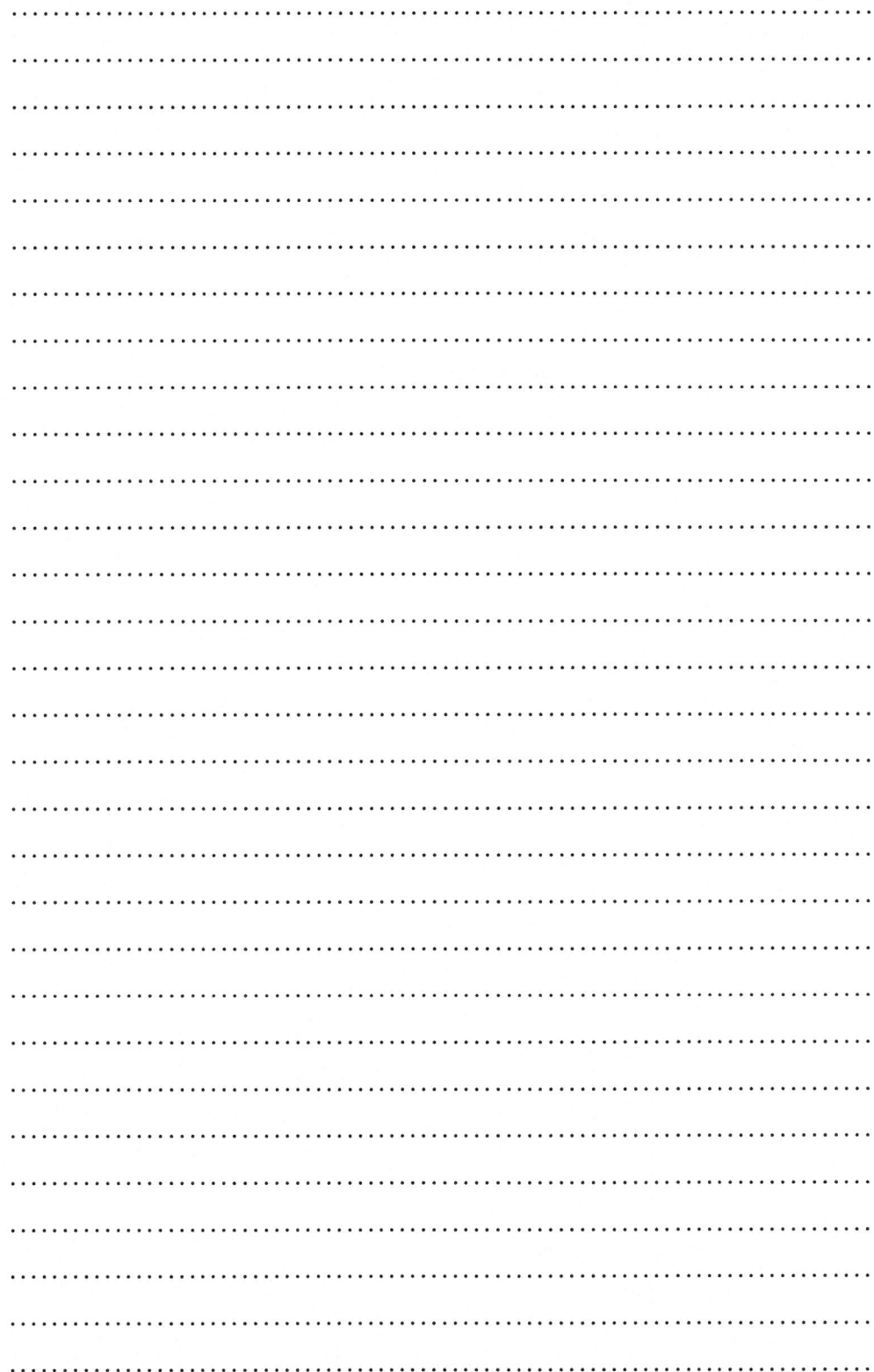

Notes + Journaling

....
....
....
....
....
....
....
....
....
....
....
....
....
....
....
....
....
....
....
....
....
....
....
....
....
....
....

Notes + Journaling

Notes + Journaling

Notes + Journaling

Notes + Journaling

Notes + Journaling

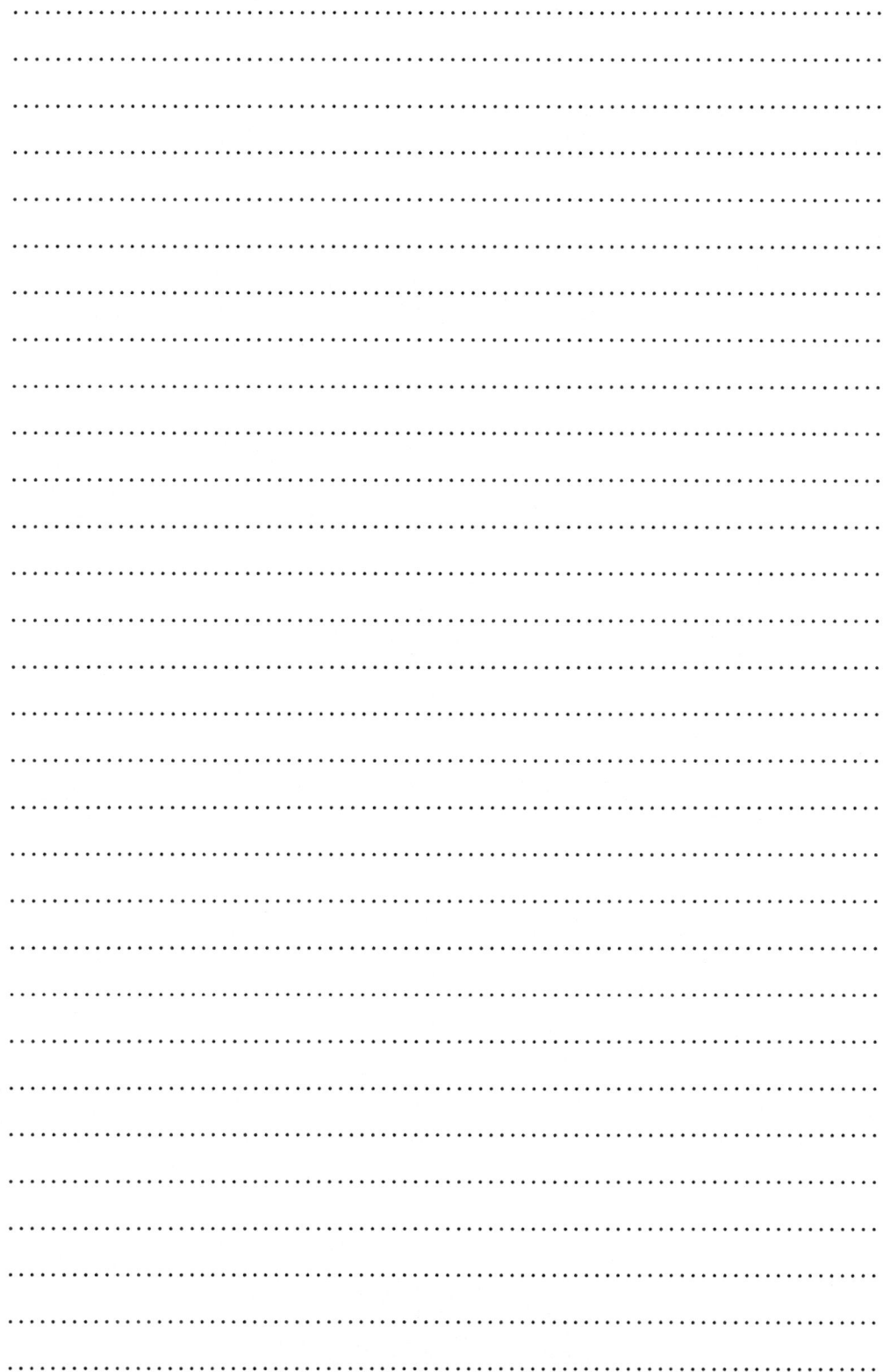

Printed in Great Britain
by Amazon